GREEN JUICING DIET

Green Juice Detox Plan for Beginners

Includes Green Smoothies and Green Juice Recipes

John Chatham

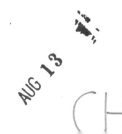

For general information on our other products and services or to obtain technical support, please contact our Customer Care Department within the U.S. at (866) 744-2665, or outside the U.S. at (510) 253-0500.

Rockridge University Press publishes its books in a variety of electronic and print formats. Some content that appears in print may not be available in electronic books, and vice versa.

ISBNs: Print 978-1-62315-054-9 | eBook 978-1-62315-055-6

TABLE OF CONTENTS

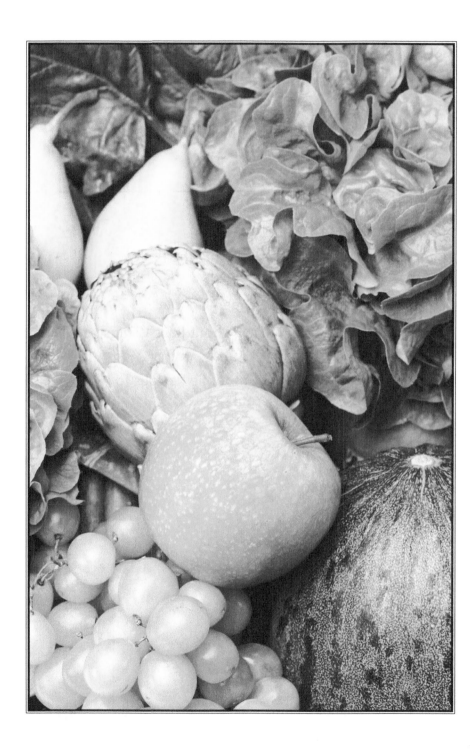

INTRODUCTION

As we learn more about the functioning of the human body, we constantly strive to find better ways to keep it healthy and make it more efficient. Naturally, we want to be free of pain and disease in order to live our lives to the fullest. We also want to look good while we do this, and as we approach health from a more holistic point of view, we're learning that how we look and feel and how we perform are all intertwined. We're also learning that we get out of our bodies what we put into them. In other words, we really are what we eat.

Now that we understand that we have much more control over disease and aging than we once believed, we are significantly more selective about what we put into our bodies. We're decreasing our intake of bad fats and simple sugars and increasing our consumption of nutrient-rich vegetables and fruits. We're also becoming aware that not all cooking methods yield the same nutritional value.

Cooking often kills healthy enzymes and damages nutrients found in raw foods, so the search is on for better ways to eat raw. After all, sitting down and eating three apples, five leaves of kale, four carrots, and a raw beet takes time that most of us don't have. This is how we ended up eating fast food (gasp!) to begin with, so what's the answer? Juicing!

In just ten or fifteen minutes, you can toss your choice of fruits and vegetables into your juicer or blender and have an entire meal's worth of nutrients in a to-go glass. The only question is where to start. Juicing can seem like a daunting task, but throughout the following pages, you'll find all you need to know about the process, plus a collection of delicious recipes to put it into practice.

Why Go Green?

There are about a thousand varieties of vegetables and fruits that you could potentially add to your juice or smoothie, so what's the big deal about the green ones? In Chapter 1, we're going to discuss what it is about these emerald-colored bits of healthful deliciousness that make them the cream of the crop. We'll also touch on the technical and nutritional differences between juices and smoothies.

Going Green

In Chapter 2, we'll answer some of the top questions that beginning juicers and smoothie makers have about the process, ranging from technical questions about the physical method of juicing, to issues regarding nutrition and health, so stick around. Chances are pretty good you'll find all the answers you need. We'll also give you thirteen helpful tips to get started, including how to choose the right produce and how to store your juice in order to preserve the most nutrients.

Blending Versus Juicing

In Chapter 3, we'll go into a bit more detail about why you may choose juicing over blending or vice versa. We'll also discuss different types of blenders and juicers to give you a better idea of what to look for when you actually go shopping. There are literally dozens of different kinds on the market, and if you search blindly, chances are pretty good you'll end up unsatisfied with the machine you purchase.

The Goods on the Greens

In order to know what produce to choose, it's a good idea to understand what each one brings to the table. In Chapter 4, we'll take a close look at the nutritional value of the top fruits and vegetables. We'll also talk about the flavors of each so you'll know how to pair it with others. As a bonus, we've thrown in a quick reference page listing each fruit and vegetable that tells you approximately how much juice it will yield.

One of the common misconceptions about green juices or smoothies is that you can only use green vegetables. We're going to debunk this myth and reveal some tasty additions that will really add zest and personality to your drink. After all, just because it's healthy doesn't mean that it has to taste bland or unpleasant!

Cleansing and Fasting

Some people just want to add green juice or a smoothie to a healthy diet in order to reap the benefits of the extra nutrients. You may also choose to go on a green juice fast or undergo a green juice cleanse to detoxify your body and cleanse your digestive tract. This isn't a good idea for everyone, but it can be extremely beneficial under the right circumstances. In Chapter 5, we'll discuss this special subset of juicing to give you a better understanding of what this is, what to expect, and whether or not this may be something you want to do.

Getting Started in Juicing

Now that you know what green juicing is and why you should try it, we're going to get you started. In the final chapter of this book, you'll learn about how consuming juices or smoothies can help you surmount various health issues, and we'll provide some great-tasting recipes to get you going.

Ready?

So enough talk—let's get to it. Why should you go green? Read on and find out!

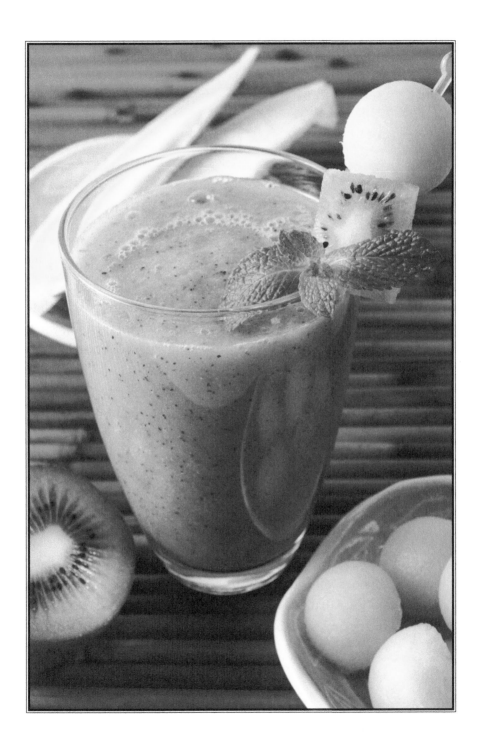

(1)

TO GREEN OR NOT TO GREEN

In today's health-conscious world, people are constantly looking for simple ways to eat a little healthier. Green juices and shakes are a great way to do that without sacrificing flavor or committing yourself to a restrictive diet. As a matter of fact, once you get the hang of it, you'll wonder why it took you so long to start juicing. This book will be your handy guide, and you'll be on your way in no time!

You may be thinking to yourself, "I can barely tolerate a few pieces of broccoli on my salad—now I'm thinking about drinking an *entire glass* of it?" Yes, you are, but don't look at it that way; if you do, you're already setting yourself up for failure. Think positively while we discuss what, exactly, green juicing is, and why you should give it a try.

What in the World Is Green Juicing?

Let's get your main misconception out of the way right out of the gate: Green juicing does *not* consist of drinking only green vegetables. You can make your juice that way if you prefer, but most people don't. Simply put, green juice is any juice (or smoothie) that is the color green. That's really all there is to it.

If you're sitting there drinking a glass of fresh green apple–green grape–kiwi juice with a splash of OJ, it's green juice. Why? Because it's *green*! Your glass may contain a concoction that's clear and bright green, a deep, rich grassy green, or maybe even more Grinch-like in hue. Your fresh-squeezed glass of deliciousness may be a rainbow of colors, but as long as there's green somewhere in that rainbow, you're drinking green juice (or a green smoothie).

Smoothies, Juices: What's the Difference?

Juices and smoothies are two extremely different animals, and though both are amazingly good for you, each has its own benefits. So what's the difference between green juice and a green smoothie? In a word: pulp.

Juice is made in a juicer, or by blending the produce and extracting the juice via cheesecloth or some other method of straining. To make a smoothie, just throw your produce into the blender and blend it all together until it reaches a drinkable consistency. Juicing is a bit more of an art form than making a smoothie, but both have some basic rules you'll need to follow for optimal results. We'll touch on those throughout the following chapters.

So what's the nutritional difference between a smoothie and a juice? Again, the answer is in the pulp. A juice without pulp has practically no fiber, so the nutrients are absorbed almost instantly. This sounds like a good thing, and if your body is used to it, it is. However, if you're new to juicing, you may experience nausea, headaches, diarrhea, or dizziness, especially if you're juice fasting and not consuming any fiber at all.

Another issue to consider when you're deciding between juices or smoothies is that the heat caused by blenders and high-speed juicers may damage the nutrients in the produce and cause oxidation, killing the beneficial live enzymes. Whether to drink juices or smoothies is just a matter of personal choice and nutritional goals. We'll explore this topic in greater depth in Chapter 3.

Did You Know? *Within fifteen minutes of consumption, your body has absorbed about 95 percent of the nutrients in a glass of pure juice. Alternatively, it takes between five and eight hours for your body to extract and absorb most of the nutrients from solid food sources.*

Green, Red, Orange, Purple: What's the Difference?

All fruits and vegetables are great for you, so what's the big deal about green juices in particular? The answer actually lies in the pigment that produces the green color: chlorophyll. Chlorophyll is often referred to as the blood of the plant and is responsible for stimulating the process known as photosynthesis. Simply stated, photosynthesis uses light to convert carbon dioxide and water into glucose, which is used for energy.

Structurally, chlorophyll is nearly identical to hemoglobin, the molecule in your blood responsible for transporting oxygen. The only difference is that the central atom of hemoglobin is iron, while that of chlorophyll is magnesium. Many people believe that chlorophyll performs the same function as hemoglobin and count this as one of its health benefits. Though not scientifically proven, it's a viable theory.

Chlorophyll also helps to replenish our red blood cells, which in turn increases oxygen levels in our blood. Other benefits often attributed to this amazing green pigment include how it:

- Promotes weight loss
- Protects DNA from damage by many carcinogens
- Enhances wound healing and tissue regeneration
- Increases energy
- Decreases inflammation in certain conditions, such as pancreatitis
- Decreases appetite because it contains the compound thylakoid

- Keeps carcinogens from attaching to DNA in many of your organs, and thus prevents development of cancer
- Helps break up calcium oxalate stones in your kidneys
- Extracts heavy metals, such as mercury, from your blood
- Stabilizes blood sugar
- Improves skin problems
- Improves mental clarity
- Maintains an alkaline environment in which diseases are unable to thrive

The reason it's better to consume chlorophyll from raw juices and smoothies rather than from cooked vegetables is that cooking lowers the chlorophyll content. You can tell when this happens because your vegetables will change from a bright green to a darker, olive green. Once they have changed to the darker hue, there is very little useful chlorophyll left in the produce.

Now that we've clarified the differences between juices and smoothies, and have reviewed the health benefits of green juices, let's move on to some of the other major juicing topics.

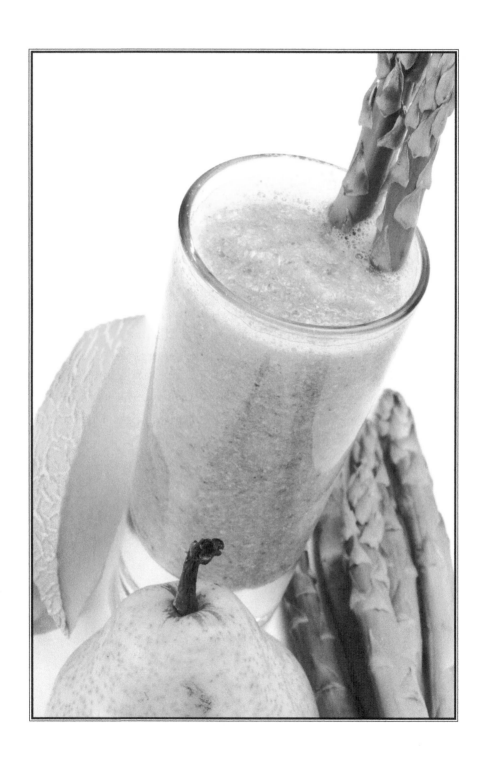

GOING GREEN: THE BASICS

I f you're like most people just starting down the mean green path, you probably have a long list of questions. This is a good thing—if you are simply throwing vegetables in a juicer or blender because you heard that it's good for you, then juicing probably isn't right for you anyway. There's a certain level of dedication required and potentially a significant financial investment, so the decision to start juicing isn't one to make lightly.

Top Ten Questions from New Juicers

Q. Why should I drink juice or make a smoothie rather than just eating my raw fruits and vegetables whole?

A. There are two main reasons why it's better to drink your vegetables: time and space. If you consider how long it would take you to eat two apples, four kale leaves, a sprig of mint, and three cups of sprouts, you'll realize how much quicker it is just to juice it.

Also, that's quite a bit of food to actually eat, so physically, it's not feasible. By juicing it, you're getting all of those nutrients in one quick, easily digestible burst! Also, what are the odds that you'll eat a huge salad without drowning it in dressing? Yet another benefit to juice or smoothies: you're skipping all of that added fat and sugar consumption.

Q. Am I limited to green vegetables only?

A. Absolutely not. Though greens should definitely be a part of your juice or smoothie, you can also use green fruits or multi-colored fruits and vegetables. The only requirement is that the juice actually be some shade of green.

Q. Can I make enough juice in the morning to get me through the day?

A. Drinking your juice immediately is definitely the best way to go, because as soon as air comes into contact with the juice, it begins to oxidize, and the nutritional value fades. That being said, drinking juice that you made three hours earlier is certainly more beneficial than a chocolate cupcake.

To keep your juice as fresh and nutritious as possible, store it in an airtight, opaque container and fill it all the way to the top so it contains as little air as possible. If you don't have enough juice to top it off, use filtered water. A little bit of lemon juice will help prevent oxidation as well. Keep the juice refrigerated until you're ready to drink it.

Q. Can I juice all fruits and vegetables?

A. Unfortunately, no. Extremely soft fruits, such as bananas, egg-plant, overripe peaches, olives, peas, beans, and avocados, are only good for smoothies, though they offer a ton of nutrients. Some people say the same about melons, but unless they're really ripe, they work just fine for juicing.

On the other end of the spectrum, extremely hard or dry produce, such as certain squashes and coconut, aren't ideal for juicing either. They're pretty hard on your juicer and don't yield much juice. Also, some seeds, such as lemon, apple, or orange seeds, are bitter.

Q. I don't really like the taste of green vegetables but really want to juice. How can I improve the taste?

A. Even people who love broccoli or beets sometimes cringe at the thought of drinking the juice. Try adding a few green grapes or a couple of apples to your cocktail. Also, some vegetables produce rich juice, so keep celery, lettuce, and cucumbers on hand, because they'll add some sweetness to your juice and lighten it up significantly. Don't be afraid to use herbs, too, such as basil and cilantro, as well as spices, such as cayenne, to add zing to your savory juices. Lemon juice adds a nice flavor snap, too.

Q. Do I need a special blender or juicer?

A. Yes, you do. We'll go into greater detail on this subject in the next chapter, but you'll need to buy a good blender if you plan on making smoothies, and a quality juicer if you want to make juice. If you're going to use grassy or leafy produce frequently, you'll need a specialized juicer for those, but it can be used for all of your juicing needs.

Q. I tried some green juice and got stomach cramps. Does that mean I can't juice?

A. Absolutely not. It's actually pretty common for green juices (or any fresh juice for that matter) to have this effect simply because your body isn't used to such a concentrated burst of nutrients. Just ease into juicing a little slower and try adding common ingredients your body is already accustomed to, like apples and celery, then work your way up in volume and originality!

Q. Why can't I just buy my juice at the supermarket?

A. There are a number of reasons why you should make your own fresh juice. To begin, packaged juices have usually been pasteurized, which means that they've been heated to kill bacteria. Many states require that juices be pasteurized prior to sale for safety reasons. The problem is that the heating process kills the beneficial enzymes and nutrients inherent to the juice.

Many store-bought juices also contain preservatives and added sugar; plus the produce was possibly treated with some form of chemical pesticides, and you have no way of knowing if it was even washed properly prior to being run through production. Finally, you don't get to create your own flavor profiles, so you're missing out on half the fun of juicing!

Q. Why is juice cleansing better than water fasting?

A. When you're juice cleansing, your body is still getting all of the nutrients it needs while cleansing and healing. Since it's receiving them without the interference of fiber, it can use the pure nutrition to heal and rejuvenate faster. Because you continue to get your nutrients with juice cleansing, you're not as prone to feel hungry, either, and you can fast for longer periods of time without worrying about starvation.

Q. Why should I limit my consumption of fruit juices?

A. While fruits are certainly good for you in small quantities, when you drink fruit juice, you're absorbing a huge shot of sugar into your bloodstream all at once. This can cause unstable blood sugar, which can lead to dizziness, and can be disastrous if you're diabetic. Many diseases, including cancer, feed on sugar, and the extra calories can cause unwanted weight gain, so take care to limit your fruit juice consumption.

Tips, Hints, and Little Secrets to Help You along Your Way

Now that we've hopefully answered some of your questions as a beginning juicer or smoothie maker, we're going to offer you some tips that will help set you on your way.

- If at all possible, buy organic produce. If it's certified organic, there won't be any chemical pesticides, hormones, or other "unnatural" chemicals that can harm you. Always wash your produce thoroughly anyway, and if you're not using organic fruits and vegetables, then you probably shouldn't eat the peels.
- If you've created a concoction that tastes absolutely disgusting, try adding cucumber, lettuce, or celery to it—these mild lifesavers may just bring your disaster back from the edge. If it seems logical to add fruit, throw an apple in, too. The apple will sweeten it up a bit and improve the palatability. Lemons are a good option as well—because they're so alkaline, lemons are great for covering up that green taste.
- Mix up your produce so you're not drinking the same fruits and vegetables all the time. Some people subscribe to the idea that

continually eating the same thing can lead to allergies, and some research supports this theory. You should change things up anyway so that you're getting a broad range of nutrients.

- Do your homework before you rush out and buy a juicer. Because there are so many options out there, it's easy to buy one that works well for you now but won't meet your needs as your juicing skills and tastes evolve. Think ahead when you make your purchase.
- The softer and riper a fruit or vegetable is, the thicker and richer the juice will be. Some fruits such as strawberries, mangos, peaches, beets, and spinach yield extremely dark, hearty juices, so you may want to combine them with lighter, milder juices, such as cucumber, carrot, or lettuce juice.
- To get the most juice out of leafy vegetables like kale, parsley, or beet greens, roll them up tightly into roll-ups or balls before you feed them through the juicer.
- Don't forget to clear the pulp catcher on your juicer frequently. Neglecting to do this will greatly reduce your juice yield and can cause spillage that will produce a sticky mess.
- Feed your juiciest produce through last so it can clean out the chute and moisten up any pulp from your dryer produce.
- If you don't have a juicer but want to make juice, you can blend your produce in the blender and then mash it through a masher or strain it through cheesecloth or a coffee filter. This is extremely messy and time consuming, but it works.
- Use your leftover pulp for muffins or stews instead of throwing it away.
- When you first start out, it's a good idea to dilute your juice with filtered water by half in order to avoid upset stomach or diarrhea. If you're fasting, this is a good way to make sure that you're getting enough water, too.

- Always take the time to clean your blender or juicer when you're finished so bacteria and mold don't start growing in it. Not only will it taint your next batch of juice, it also can make you really sick.
- Have fun and experiment! This is a new adventure that will keep you healthy and happy for years to come. Discover flavors you love and don't be afraid to try new combinations. You never know what you'll like until you try it!

If you follow these simple tips and use a bit of common sense, you'll be making delicious, healthy juices and smoothies in no time. You'll surely come up with a few "yucks," but as your palate progresses, you'll get a feel for what works well together and what doesn't. And remember, just because your friend loves a certain combination doesn't mean that you'll be jumping for joy over that flavor, too.

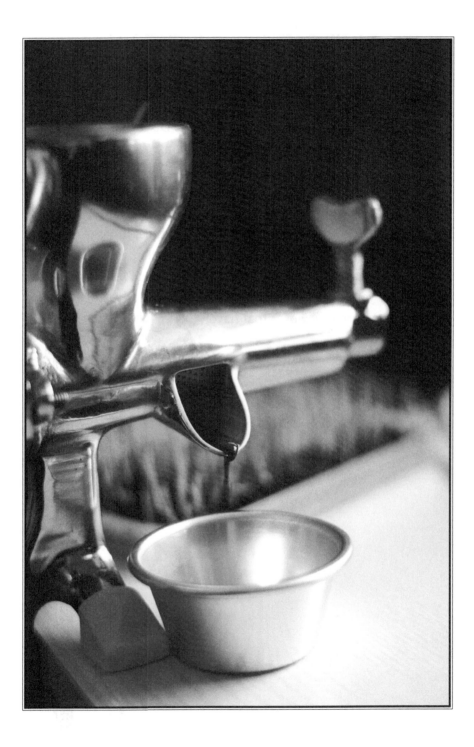

$$\bigcirc\!\!3$$

BLENDER OR JUICER: PICKING THE PERFECT MACHINE FOR YOUR NEEDS

Deciding whether to juice or blend is a choice that depends upon what you want to achieve. If you just want to add some nutrients to your diet along with some fiber, then blending will suit your needs perfectly. If your goal is quick absorption of large amounts of nutrients, or if you want to undergo a cleansing experience, then juicing is the way to go. Here are a few more points to consider when making your decision:

- Juicing requires very little digestion, so if you are experiencing problems with fiber (due to illness or otherwise), then juice is the best way to increase your nutrients without stressing your digestive tract.
- Smoothies require additional digestion to extract the nutrients from the plant fibers, but the fiber helps with elimination on its way out.
- Juicing is a more concentrated, rapid source of nutrients, because the nutrients are readily available, and you can drink much more because there's no fiber to fill you up.

- If you're one of those people who hate to eat green vegetables, then juicing is a great way to get all of your daily nutrients in just a few swallows.
- Some professionals postulate that the chewing action required by food is a necessary part of the digestive process, so according to that theory, if you're drinking a chunky smoothie that requires a bit of jaw action, you may be taking the healthier route.
- If your goal is a complete cleanse, fiber is usually discouraged so the body can use the energy it saves from the digestive process to heal and cleanse, thus making juice the best option.

When it comes right down to it, the decision to drink juices or smoothies (or a combination of the two) depends upon your goals. If you're healthy and just want to add some extra nutrients into your diet, then smoothies are a great idea. If you don't like the texture of ground fruits and veggies, are short on time, or want the extra burst of nutrients without feeling full, then you may prefer juice. As with all decisions about your body, do your research and make an educated choice based upon what's personally best for you.

Whether you're making a juice or a smoothie, you're going to need a good piece of equipment to take your produce from chewable to drinkable. There are dozens of different blenders and juicers on the market, and what kind you need depends upon a few different variables, including:

- How often are you going to use it?
- What are you going to be blending or juicing?
- How many people are you using it for?
- How much space do you have?
- How quiet do you need it to be?
- How much money do you have to spend?

Since there aren't quite as many factors that go into buying a blender as a juicer, and you can get one for a fairly decent price (usually under $100), let's review the blender choices first.

What to Look for in a Blender

A blender is a blender, right? Wrong. There are as many different blenders out there as there are things to put in them. The choices can be overwhelming, and there are some things to watch out for that you might not consider as a first-time buyer. That's why we've gone to longtime smoothie makers to find out what problems they've encountered, to ensure that you avoid those pitfalls on your journey to the perfect smoothie. Here are a few of the top tips that should help you on your way:

- Try to stick with metal blades and internal parts, avoiding plastic, especially if you're going to be using your blender frequently.
- Anything under 500 watts probably won't be effective.
- Choose a blender with at least two different speed settings, plus a pulse function, because it's best to start on low to chop, then work your way up through the speeds to get the finest consistency with the least amount of nutrient-killing heat.
- Look for products with warranties, and buy your blender from stores that stand behind their products. It's frustrating to invest good money in a blender just to have it break two weeks later, only to find out that the company or store won't stand behind the product.

Blenders range in price from about $20 to well over $500, but there's really no need to go to the top for a machine that meets your needs. That being said, a $20 blender probably won't do the job, at least not for very long. If you're serious about making smoothies, it's best to invest in a good blender that will last, rather than buying several cheap blenders over time that continue to break—and have no warranty.

Some Good "Smoothie Blender" Suggestions

A few excellent choices broken down by price include:

$300+ Range: The best in form and function

- **Vitamix 5200:** 1000 watts, powerful 2 HP motor, 64-ounce carafe, 7-year warranty, BPA-free carafe, variable speed dial as well as the ability to pulse, plus a patented tamper so you can quickly blend even thick ingredients.
- **Blendtec Home Pro Choice Total Blender:** 1500 watts, 3 HP motor, 64-ounce carafe, lifetime warranty on blade and coupling, 3-year warranty on base, 29K RPM, 6 blending options plus pulse. Features Smart-Touch Tec-nology© that automatically speeds up and slows down as necessary and shuts off at the end of the cycle.

$200–$300 Range: Top quality

- **Breville 800BLXL Hemisphere:** 1000 watts, 67-ounce polycarbonate carafe, uniquely shaped carafe, blades that allow for zero dead space around the edge of the carafe, 1-year limited warranty, 2 speeds plus pulse.
- **Cuisinart CBT 100 PowerEdge:** 1000 watts, 1.3 HP motor, BPA-free carafe, 3-year limited warranty, high and low settings plus preprogrammed smoothie, pulse, and ice-crush settings that intermittently speed up and slow down for best results.

$100–$200 Range: Very effective

- **KitchenAid KSB560MC Blender:** 720 watts, 0.9 HP motor, 56-ounce polycarbonate carafe, 1-year replacement warranty, 5 speeds plus pulse.

Under $100: Great value for the price
- **Oster Beehive:** 600 watts, 40-ounce glass carafe, 1-year warranty, 2 speeds plus pulse.

More expensive isn't always better, but in the case of these blenders, you really don't want to go with anything under $50. Most likely you'll just be wasting your money on a product that's not going to work well and will only break within a few months. Spend the extra money and do it right!

What Type of Juicer Is Right for You?

Most of us have used a blender at some point in our lives, so purchasing one isn't completely alien territory. When it comes to juicers, however, it's like learning a whole new language. They often look awkward, and figuring out exactly what all of those pieces are for is an exercise in physics. Yet there's no need to feel intimidated; we're going to clear up any confusion and give you a preliminary sense of what to look for on your search.

Did You Know? *Juicers come in six basic styles: centrifugal, masticating, upright masticating, twin gear (aka triturating), wheatgrass, and hydraulic press.*

Buying a juicer can be a major investment, so knowing the facts about the equipment prior to making your purchase is only smart. Each type of juicer is great at producing the juice for which it's been specialized, but buying one that doesn't meet your overall needs can be an expensive, messy mistake. Let's break these down and discuss the pros and cons of each.

- **Centrifugal Juicers** are the least expensive juicers on the market and the type that most department stores carry. They extract your juice by shredding the produce and then using centrifugal force to spin the pulp against a strainer at extremely high RPMs. This is OK if you're juicing soft produce, but these machines produce much more waste (wet pulp) than other types of juicers.

  Pros: Speed and affordability.

  Cons: Low efficiency (high waste); decreased shelf life, because the extraction process spins oxidizing air into the juice; and difficulty juicing grasses or leafy produce.

- **Masticating Juicers** extract juice by literally "chewing" the food using a single auger or gear and then separating the juice as it chews. This process results in more nutrients, fiber, and enzymes being extracted from the pulp because of the chewing action.

  Pros: Greater efficiency, less air in the juice, more nutrients extracted from the produce, and less nutrients lost due to heat or oxidization, because it operates at a lower RPM than a centrifugal juicer. Also, masticating juicers often do a good job with leafy greens and grasses. Many masticating juicers also homogenize your produce, so you can make baby foods, ice cream, sauces, or nut butters.

  Cons: Higher cost, larger size, and more noise. A masticating juicer also takes significantly more time than a centrifugal juicer does.

- **Upright Masticating Juicers** have all of the benefits of a typical, single-auger masticating juicer but are designed to operate in an upright position in order to be more space-efficient. There are also a couple of design differences. Instead of being chewed and extracted, the juice is squeezed out first, then the pulp is crushed and pressed again in a second phase to extract even more juice.

Pros: Higher juice yield and less waste, a smaller space requirement, and less waste due to heat or injected air. They can capably juice just about anything.

Cons: Significantly higher cost, and they're often noisy.

- **Triturating (Twin Gear) Juicers** extract juice in much the same manner as a masticating juicer, except that they squeeze the pulp between two interlocking gears. Because they're designed to be slow and powerful, these juicers crack the nutrients from the cells, so not only do you get a higher yield of juice, you get more nutrients, too. Triturating juicers are typically the most expensive juicer, but because you can do so many things with them and they produce so little waste, they're worth it if you can swing the cost.

  Pros: The higher juice/nutrient yield, less waste from either heat production or the extraction process, the ability to efficiently juice grasses and leaves, and the capability of the machine to homogenize in order to make baby foods, nut butters, ice creams, sorbets, and even pastas.

  Cons: High cost, greater space requirements, and more time due to slower RPMs.

- **Wheatgrass Juicers** do exactly what the name implies: juice grasses. They aren't designed to juice anything other than grasses, with the possible exception of a few small, soft fruits, such as grapes. These juicers come in both manual and electric styles.

  Pros: The fact that you can get an efficient, affordable model if all you're looking to do is make a nice green shot for health reasons or to add to a recipe.

  Cons: It's an expensive piece of equipment given its specialized, limited capabilities, and the fact that they're often bulky. Especially considering that most decent juicers can handle leafy greens and grasses, this isn't a necessary piece of equipment for green juicing anymore if you buy a suitable standard juicer.

- **Hydraulic Press Juicers** also known as Norwalk Juicers, extract juice in the most efficient way possible: they literally press it out. There's no chewing or grinding of the produce, and there's extremely little waste. Also, since it's a simple pressing process, there's no heat produced, or air forced into the juice. It's far and away the best way to extract juice.

  Pros: Practically no waste, no damage to the juice, and no air pressed in to cause oxidation.

  Cons: Extremely expensive at around $2,500 and take up a large amount of space—great if you have the room and the money, but unrealistic for most of us.

Choosing the right juicer or blender is an important part of your experience, so educate yourself about your options and choose wisely. Because there are so many different brands, and people juice for so many reasons, it's difficult to make specific product recommendations, so just pay attention to what the various machines offer and match those features to what you intend to use most.

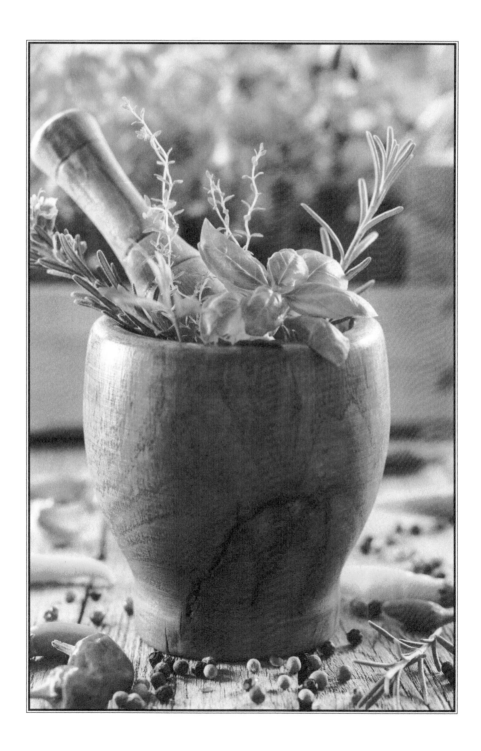

4

WHAT ARE THOSE GREEN GOODIES?

Getting the hang of juicing requires a certain amount of flavor savvy that you can develop only through personal experience, as everyone's tastes are somewhat different. What you may consider delicious may be repulsive to your neighbor, so trial and error here will truly be your best friend. But first, we'll give you a few pointers, so you're not going in totally blind. With this list and a little bit of common sense, your juicing journey won't be quite so dangerous to your palate!

The Green Juice Ratio for Success: *The easiest way to remember how to mix your green juice in order to keep a palatable flavor, at least in the beginning, is to follow the 4-3-2-1 method. Use 4 parts sweet juice, such as apple, grape, or pineapple; 3 parts grassy greens, such as wheatgrass, sprouts, spinach, or lettuce; 2 parts tangy juice, such as lemon, lime, or kiwi; and 1 part spicy or zesty juice or powder, such as mint, cayenne, or ginger. Of course, if you like savory juices, feel free to eliminate the sweet element!*

The Great Green List

Since we've already discussed the fact that green juices don't have to be prepared entirely with green produce, this list isn't going to be green-only either. Instead, we'll cover many of the green fruits and veggies to include in your juice as well as herbs, spices, and deliciously nutritious produce of other colors, too.

By the end of this chapter, you'll understand how much juice to expect from each ingredient as well as its flavor profile, health benefits, and nutritional content. To make your experience even easier, we're going to break each item down into the flavor profiles described in the 4-3-2-1 method, starting with sweet and working our way down to spicy. When discussing yields, we'll speak in terms of weight instead of by the piece, in order to keep as accurate as possible.

Did You Know? *Though each fruit, vegetable, and herb is different, and some juicers are more efficient than others, a good rule of thumb is that one pound of produce yields about one cup of juice.*

Naturally Sweet

These fruits and vegetables contain natural sweetness and will probably be the easiest for your body to get habituated to as you begin juicing. If you're having problems adapting to drinking your nutrients, try adding a few more of these to your blender or juicer until you adjust to the grassier or earthier flavors of some of your greener or less traditional ingredients.

Apples

- **Color:** Green

- **Yield:** 1 pound = ¾ to 1 cup juice

- **Flavor Profile:** Sweet with just a bit of tartness

- **Health Benefits:** Apples are rich in phytonutrients, called polyphenols, as well as antioxidants. They help regulate blood sugar, decrease your risk of asthma, and reduce your odds of developing several types of cancer, including lung, colon, and breast cancers.

Apricots

- **Color:** Peach

- **Yield:** 1 pound = ½ to ¾ cup juice

- **Flavor Profile:** Moderately sweet, sometimes a little tart, musky, and mildly "peachy"

- **Health Benefits:** Rich in beta-carotene and vitamins A and C, apricots help fight free radicals that cause eye conditions such as macular degeneration. They may also help you maintain healthy levels of HDL, the "good" cholesterol.

Beets

- **Color:** Deep red

- **Yield:** 1 pound = ¾ to 1 cup juice

- **Flavor Profile:** Sweet and earthy

- **Health Benefits:** Beets are truly a superfood that almost deserve their own book to cover their many amazing health benefits! They're a great source of beta-carotene, phytonutrients, manganese, and vitamin C, and they help keep your heart, eyes, and nerves healthy.

Betalain, an incredibly powerful antioxidant and anti-inflammatory unique to beets, plays a major role in cellular detoxification. Plus the combination of antioxidants, nutrients, and anti-inflammatories help protect you from prostate, lung, stomach, colon, testicular, and nerve cancers.

Blackberries or Raspberries

- **Color:** Black or red

- **Yield:** 1 pound = 1 cup juice

- **Flavor Profile:** Rich, sweet, and sometimes a bit tart

- **Health Benefits:** Two more examples of health superstars, blackberries and raspberries are rich in the phytonutrients called tannins, as well as copper, folate, magnesium, manganese, potassium, and vitamins C, E, and K. They're also a good source of omega-3 fatty acids, which help keep your brain and heart healthy.

The antioxidants in these berries protect you from a host of diseases, including cancer and heart disease. They also fight free radicals and help prevent signs of aging, including wrinkles, dull skin, and muscle loss. The antimicrobial properties help keep you free of digestive issues, too, as well as fungal infections, such as yeast infections.

Cantaloupes

- **Color:** Yellow-orange

- **Yield:** 1 pound = 1 to 1½ cups juice

- **Flavor Profile:** Sweet, musky, and refreshing

- **Health Benefits:** Chock full of such nutrients and antioxidants as beta-carotene, folate, potassium, magnesium, and vitamins A, B1, B6, C, and K, cantaloupe not only adds a delicious sweetness to your juice, it also protects you from a host of agues and illnesses, including macular degeneration, emphysema, fatigue, irregular blood sugar, low metabolism, stroke, heart disease, immune weakness, and several types of cancer.

Carrots

- **Color:** Bright orange

- **Yield:** 1 pound = 1 to 1¼ cups juice

- **Flavor Profile:** Sweet and mild

- **Health Benefits:** Like cantaloupe, the health benefits of carrots are off the charts and would take an entire chapter to cover in full. They're a great source of vitamin A, beta-carotene, the entire B complex of vitamins, calcium, manganese, molybdenum, phosphorus, and potassium. The nutrients, antioxidants, and anti-inflammatory properties help maintain eye health and promote good cardiovascular health. They also help protect you from cancer, as well as prevent signs of aging, and do wonders for your hair, nails, and skin.

Cranberries

- **Color:** Red

- **Yield:** 1 pound = ½ to ¾ cup juice

- **Flavor Profile:** Mildly sweet and tart

- **Health Benefits:** Most people know that cranberries are great for your kidneys, but the red color also tells us that cranberries are full of antioxidants, and they have anti-inflammatory properties, too. Nutrients include manganese, the antioxidant and anti-aging kingpin resveratrol and vitamins C, E, and K.

  They help prevent numerous health problems, including periodontal disease, kidney infections and stones, urinary tract infections, arterial plaque buildup and heart disease, and signs of aging such as wrinkles and thinning skin. Finally, cranberries may actually help reduce your downtime from colds and the flu.

Grapes

- **Color:** Green

- **Yield:** 1 pound = ¾ to 1 cup juice

- **Flavor Profile:** Sweet and tart

- **Health Benefits:** Chock full of antioxidants (about thirty in total!), manganese, potassium, and vitamins C, B1, B6, and K, grapes help protect you from breast, colon, and prostate cancers, cardiovascular disease, irregular blood sugar levels, and cognitive decline.

Honeydews

- **Color:** Green

- **Yield:** 1 pound = 1 to 1¼ cups juice

- **Flavor Profile:** Sweet and light

- **Health Benefits:** Honeydew is a good source of vitamin A, potassium, vitamin C, copper, and B vitamins, including niacin and thiamin. Honeydew is great for helping your body detoxify, and also protects you from cardiovascular disease, infection, skin damage caused by oxidation and collagen loss, several types of cancer, and eye disorders like macular degeneration.

Kiwifruits

- **Color:** Green

- **Yield:** 1 pound = 1 to 1½ cups juice

- **Flavor Profile:** Sweet and tart

- **Health Benefits:** Kiwis actually have more vitamin C than oranges, as well as calcium and a host of vitamins and minerals. They have some amazing benefits, such as helping to lower your blood pressure, promoting circulatory health, protecting your DNA from oxidation, and reducing the risk of respiratory issues, especially in children.

Oranges

- **Color:** Orange

- **Yield:** 1 pound = ¾ to 1 cup juice

- **Flavor Profile:** Sweet, zesty, and sometimes a bit tart

- **Health Benefits:** You probably already know that oranges are a great source of vitamin C, but did you know that they also have calcium, folate, potassium, vitamins A and B1, and several different phytonutrients, including anthocyanins, flavanones, polyphenols, and hydroxycinnamic acids? Oranges help lower blood pressure, fight off colds and the flu, and protect you from diseases such as lung and stomach cancers, arthritis, and atherosclerosis. In addition, they reduce your risk of stroke and heart disease.

Papayas

- **Color:** Orange

- **Yield:** 1 pound = ¾ to 1 cup juice

- **Flavor Profile:** Mildly sweet, musky, and earthy

- **Health Benefits:** Though this brightly colored fruit is a bit of an acquired taste, the health benefits are well worth the adjustment. Papayas have a ton of vitamin C and are rich in vitamin A, beta-carotene, folic acid, pantothenic acids, folate, potassium, magnesium, and vitamins E and B. They promote heart health, good vision, and a healthy immune system. Papayas also help prevent colon cancer, arthritis, and asthma.

Pears

- **Color:** Translucent green

- **Yield:** 1 pound = ¾ to 1 cup juice

- **Flavor Profile:** Mildly sweet, light, and a bit rustic

- **Health Benefits:** Pears have phytonutrients and are a great source of vitamin C and vitamin K. Pears are more easily tolerated by people with food allergies, and they promote good eye health. Vitamin K is used by your body for effective blood clotting and to maintain bone health.

Pineapples

- **Color:** Yellow

- **Yield:** 1 pound = ¾ to 1 cup juice

- **Flavor Profile:** Sweet, fruity, and tropical

- **Health Benefits:** Pineapple contains the enzyme bromelain as well as manganese, copper, folate, and vitamins B6 and C, which help keep your immune system strong and assist in digestive, eye, and heart health. Pineapples are also a great source of energy because of the sugars and B6. The bromelain is an anti-inflammatory that helps protect you from arthritis, cancers, and other inflammation-related diseases.

Pomegranates

- **Color:** Pink

- **Yield:** 1 pound = ½ to ¾ cup juice

- **Flavor Profile:** Sweet, rich, and reminiscent of grape juice

- **Health Benefits:** Pomegranates provide a healthy dose of vitamins C and B5 as well as potassium, flavonoids, and other natural phenols and polyphenols that act as powerful antioxidants. Adding pomegranate juice to your green juice or smoothie can help protect you from several different types of cancer, heart disease, atherosclerosis, mental decline, kidney disease, and diabetes.

Strawberries

- **Color:** Red-pink

- **Yield:** 1 pound = ½ to ¾ cup juice

- **Flavor Profile:** Sweet and nectar-like

- **Health Benefits:** Like other berries, strawberries are packed with antioxidants as well as vitamin C, potassium, vitamin K, magnesium, iodine, and omega-3 fatty acids. They're great for heart health, including prevention of atherosclerosis, and they help maintain normal blood sugar levels, as well as protecting you from colon, esophageal, and breast cancers. They can also keep you looking and feeling young by preventing cognitive decline, macular degeneration, arthritis, and digestive issues.

Sweet Potatoes

- **Color:** Orange

- **Yield:** 1 pound = ½ cup juice

- **Flavor Profile:** Sweet and earthy

- **Health Benefits:** Sweet potatoes are packed with vitamins A, C, and B complex, potassium, copper, manganese, and tryptophan. These sweetly flavored, richly colored tubers are, in fact, even better for your eyes than carrots while also helping to protect you from such illnesses as heart disease, diabetes, nervous system disorders, and hemophilia.

Did You Know? *Sweet potatoes contain nearly 440 percent of your recommended daily amount of vitamin A in a single serving. Throw some cinnamon in and you have a disease-fighting powerhouse of a drink!*

Watermelons

- **Color:** Pink

- **Yield:** 1 pound = 1 to 1½ cups juice

- **Flavor Profile:** Sweet, light, and refreshing

- **Health Benefits:** Watermelon is largely water, so it yields a considerable amount of juice. It's rich in potassium, magnesium, and lycopene, which makes it great for your eyes. It also contains vitamins A and C, and it can help prevent breast, colon, endometrial, lung, prostate, and rectal cancers. It gives you a nice energy boost and helps keep you looking and feeling young because of the amino acid arginine. Finally, watermelon helps you avoid high blood pressure, type 2 diabetes, and erectile dysfunction.

Green, Grassy, and Fresh

Once you get the hang of juicing and your palate adjusts to the textural difference of drinking your produce in addition to eating it, you'll start appreciating the subtle differences that each fruit or vegetable can add. The grassy flavors of some greens may be too much for you at first—if so, just add in some cucumber or apple juice. If you want to go hardcore green, start with some of the lighter-flavored produce until your body adjusts to the delicious green freshness.

Alfalfa

- **Color:** Green

- **Yield:** 1 pound = ⅔ to 1 cup juice

- **Flavor Profile:** Earthy but extremely mild

- **Health Benefits:** Alfalfa is considered the richest land source of minerals because the roots go down thirty feet deep in search of minerals. It boasts vitamins C, E, A, K, B1, and B6, as well as calcium, carotene, protein, iron, potassium, and zinc; it is also an anti-inflammatory and antioxidant. Alfalfa helps get rid of kidney problems in addition to assisting with arthritis, digestive issues, high cholesterol, urinary problems, and an entire array of other ailments. In other words—drink it!

Artichokes

- **Color:** Green

- **Yield:** 1 pound = $\frac{2}{3}$ to 1 cup juice

- **Flavor Profile:** Strong, earthy, and sometimes a little bitter

- **Health Benefits:** Artichokes are one of those foods that many people just don't bother with because they're somewhat exotic and awkward to work with, but they have some truly incredible health benefits that make this leafy little vegetable well worth your time. They're rich in cancer- and disease-fighting antioxidants (eight different ones, more than any other vegetable) and have actually been shown to cause apoptosis (cell death) in leukemia, prostate cancer, and breast cancer. Artichokes may even reduce your chance of developing breast cancer to begin with.

  They are also excellent for digestion and the health of your liver—as a matter of fact, studies show they may actually promote liver tissue regeneration. They are a natural diuretic, so they're good for your kidneys, too.

> **Did You Know?** *Some people prefer to lightly parboil the artichoke prior to juicing in order to get the most out of it. If you choose to parboil, take care to do so lightly; otherwise you'll destroy its nutritious enzymes and nutrients.*

Asparagus

- **Color:** Green

- **Yield:** 1 pound = ¾ to 1 cup juice

- **Flavor Profile:** Green and rich

- **Health Benefits:** Asparagus is a great source of both vitamins and minerals and even contains protein. Just some of the nutrients found in this crisp delicacy include phosphorus, potassium, manganese, molybdenum, choline, selenium, calcium, and magnesium, as well as vitamins A, C, E, K, and B complex.

  Asparagus contains several antioxidants, has anti-inflammatory properties, and is proven to lower your chances of developing colon cancer, Lou Gehrig's disease, cardiovascular disease, and type 2 diabetes. It also helps with digestive health, because it contains the carbohydrate inulin, which promotes absorption of nutrients in your large intestine.

Barley Grass

- **Color:** Green

- **Yield:** 1 pound = ¾ to 1 cup juice

- **Flavor Profile:** Grassy

- **Health Benefits:** Barley grass contains four times the amount of calcium as a glass of milk, and as much protein as one ounce of steak. It also has about twenty times more iron than spinach does and is rich in vitamins A, C, E, K, and B complex. It has every amino acid that your body requires and is great for those trying to lose weight or get a good night's sleep.

  Since it has so many antioxidants, it helps protect you from numerous conditions, including cancer, heart disease, cognitive decline, and digestive issues. Finally, it helps protect against signs of aging and alkalizes the body so that your immune system functions well and diseases such as cancer are unable to thrive.

Bell Peppers

- **Color:** Green for the chlorophyll, though all colors have amazing health benefits

- **Yield:** 1 pound = 1 to 1¼ cups juice

- **Flavor Profile:** Sweet, green, and mildly peppery

- **Health Benefits:** Peppers boast significant quantities of phytonutrients and antioxidants as well as vitamins and minerals, including vitamins A, C, E, K, and B complex, magnesium, potassium, and manganese. They also have anti-inflammatory properties that protect you from several types of cancer, including digestive cancers, and such diseases as arthritis, heart disease, and atherosclerosis. The beta-carotene in peppers helps keep your eyes healthy, too.

Broccoli

- **Color:** Green

- **Yield:** 1 pound = ¾ to 1 cup juice

- **Flavor Profile:** Extremely rich and green

- **Health Benefits:** Broccoli has nearly every vitamin and major mineral as well as protein. It's actually got about as much calcium as a glass of milk, and is packed with phytonutrients that help support detox at every single stage, starting at the DNA level.

  Because it's so rich in antioxidants and is also an anti-inflammatory, broccoli helps protect you from several types of cancer, such as bladder, breast, colon, and ovarian cancers. Finally, the beta-carotene in broccoli protects you from such eye diseases as macular degeneration and cataracts.

Celery

- **Color:** Light green

- **Yield:** 1 pound = 1 to 1¼ cups juice

- **Flavor Profile:** Light, refreshing, slightly peppery

- **Health Benefits:** It's not just a great partner to blue cheese—celery is a good source of vitamins A, B, C, and K, as well as potassium, manganese, calcium, magnesium, and tryptophan. It's been used for centuries as a natural diuretic, and also promotes arterial health, lowers your bad cholesterol, and helps keep your immune system strong by protecting you from free radicals.

Did You Know? *Because of its mild, familiar flavor, celery—along with cucumber—works as a great base for just about any juice.*

Chard

- **Color:** Dark green

- **Yield:** 1 pound = 1 cup juice

- **Flavor Profile:** Grassy and mildly sweet

- **Health Benefits:** The leaves of chard are packed with phytonutrients, calcium, vitamins A, B complex, C, and K, iron, manganese, sodium, potassium, and copper. It's great for protecting you from anemia, osteoporosis, heart disease, cardiovascular disease, prostate and colon cancers, arthritis, cognitive decline, Alzheimer's disease, and high cholesterol. In addition, it gives your immune system a real boost. These are just a few of the multitude of benefits you obtain from adding chard to your juice.

Collard, Dandelion, Mustard, and Turnip Greens

- **Color:** Deep green

- **Yield:** 1 pound = 1 cup juice

- **Flavor Profile:** Grassy and earthy

- **Health Benefits:** These greens are packed with calcium, vitamins A and K, and omega-3 fatty acids, and contain lesser amounts of practically every vitamin and mineral. The large array of antioxidants serve to protect you from the signs of aging, cancer, heart disease, and other diseases caused by the inflammatory effects of free radicals. Greens also help keep your blood pressure normal, and the high amounts of calcium and vitamin K promote bone health, protecting you from osteoporosis and arthritis.

Did You Know? *When you're preparing your carrots, radishes, celery, beets, and other root vegetables, don't you dare throw away those green tops! They're packed with many of the same nutrients—chlorophyll, too—as the vegetable to which they're attached! Toss 'em into the juicer instead of the compost bin.*

Cucumbers

- **Color:** Light green

- **Yield:** 1 pound = 1 to 1½ cups juice

- **Flavor Profile:** Light, mildly sweet, and refreshing

- **Health Benefits:** Rich in phytonutrients, antioxidants, and vitamin K, cucumbers are a great base for almost any juice, whether you're using vegetables or fruits. They help protect you from cancer and other damage and diseases caused by free radicals, and they also contain lignans, which may help protect you from estrogen-related cancers such as breast, prostate, ovarian, and uterine cancers. Plus, cucurbitacins, which are unique to cucumbers, block signaling pathways that some cancer cells need to grow.

Kale

- **Color:** Dark green

- **Yield:** 1 pound = 1 cup juice

- **Flavor Profile:** Rich and grassy

- **Health Benefits:** As with other leafy greens, kale is rich in calcium, vitamins, minerals, and antioxidants. It's great for detox support at all levels and helps prevent many forms of cancer as well as other diseases and ailments caused by free radicals. The anti-inflammatory properties protect you from heart disease and atherosclerosis, and the calcium and vitamin K work together to keep your bones strong.

Kohlrabi

- **Color:** Green

- **Yield:** 1 pound = ¾ to 1 cup juice

- **Flavor Profile:** Extremely rich and leafy

- **Health Benefits:** Kohlrabi, like other leafy green vegetables, contains calcium, a wide array of vitamins and minerals, and large amounts of chlorophyll. It's a common ingredient in weight loss juices, and it's excellent for skin conditions such as eczema.

Loose Leaf, Butter, and Romaine Lettuces

- **Color:** Light to dark green, depending upon variety

- **Yield:** 1 pound = 1 cup juice

- **Flavor Profile:** Light and refreshing, and grassy with the greener lettuces

- **Health Benefits:** The greener a lettuce leaf is, the more chlorophyll and other phytonutrients it contains. Lettuces are packed with vitamin A and carotenes, which are fantastic for your eyes and skin. They also protect you from lung and mouth cancers.

The vitamin K helps with bone growth and strength and it fights off Alzheimer's, too. The folates and vitamin C are powerful anti-oxidants that fight free radicals. Lettuces are also a good source of minerals, such as magnesium, iron, calcium and potassium, which help your body maintain a healthy metabolism.

Potatoes

- **Color:** Milky

- **Yield:** 1 pound = ⅔ to 1 cup juice

- **Flavor Profile:** Light and mildly earthy

- **Health Benefits:** White potatoes are known in the juicing world for their efficiency in clearing up acne and other skin blemishes. With the exception of vitamin A, they also contain nearly every vitamin, especially vitamins C and B6, potassium, iron, and copper. A special note about the vitamin C: You really only reap its benefit when you eat a potato raw or in fresh juice, because it's lost during the cooking process. Potatoes help support your immune system, promote heart health, work to keep your blood pressure low, and help maintain your electrolyte balance.

Spinach

- **Color:** Dark green

- **Yield:** 1 pound = ½ to 1 cup juice

- **Flavor Profile:** Rich, grassy, and pungent

- **Health Benefits:** Spinach shares the same health benefits and nutrients as other leafy greens and is also extremely rich in iron, which helps keep your blood healthy. Popeye wasn't wrong when he said to eat your spinach—it helps keep your bones strong, your muscles functioning well, and prevents several types of cancers. In addition, it's rich in chlorophyll and antioxidants.

Did you know? *Spinach contains a whopping 247 percent of your daily recommended intake of vitamin A, which is a super-antioxidant that helps with everything from cancer prevention to fighting the signs of aging.*

Spirulina

- **Color:** Bright green

- **Yield:** 1 pound = ¾ cup juice

- **Flavor Profile:** Extremely grassy and strong

- **Health Benefits:** This blue-green algae turns your drink a bright green and packs an amazing 60 percent vegetable protein. It's also a great source of iron, zinc, magnesium, copper, calcium, and vitamins E and C. It has quality beta-carotene and gamma linolenic acid, an essential fatty acid. Spirulina is excellent for helping protect you from cancers, heart disease, gastric disorders, inflammatory disorders, and other diseases caused by free radicals.

Sprouts

- **Color:** White

- **Yield:** 1 pound = ½ to ¾ cup juice

- **Flavor Profile:** Light with almost no flavor, making them great as a base for more pungent greens

- **Health Benefits:** A good source of vitamins C and B complex, sprouts are rich in antioxidants and help keep your body alkaline, which deters cancer growth.

Summer Squash

- **Color:** Yellow

- **Yield:** 1 pound = ¾ cup juice

- **Flavor Profile:** Light and earthy

- **Health Benefits:** Summer squash provides a great source of vitamins A, C, K, and B complex, as well as lutein and zeaxanthin, which protect your eyes from disorders such as macular degeneration and cataracts. It also contains omega-3 fatty acids, manganese, phosphorus, magnesium, tryptophan, potassium, and zinc, promoting cardiovascular, heart, digestive, and prostate health, as well as helping to stabilize your blood sugar. Finally, the antioxidants and anti-inflammatory properties in summer squash assist in preventing cancer.

Wheatgrass

- **Color:** Green

- **Yield:** 1 pound = ¾ to 1 cup juice

- **Flavor Profile:** Grassy and rich

- **Health Benefits:** Wheatgrass is rich in chlorophyll and the nutrients found in the other types of grass. It helps to boost your energy, stabilize your blood sugar, and is great for detoxification and healing.

Spicy

Arugula

- **Color:** Dark green

- **Yield:** 1 pound = ½ to 1 cup juice

- **Flavor Profile:** Peppery and fresh

- **Health Benefits:** Arugula has the same health benefits as other lettuces but adds a pleasant, naturally peppery flavor to your juice, while helping you detoxify and fight disease.

Cabbage

- **Color:** Green to milky

- **Yield:** 1 pound = 1 cup juice

- **Flavor Profile:** Pungent and spicy

- **Health Benefits:** Cabbage is another superfood offering a range of benefits from cancer prevention to weight loss. It's used to treat ulcers and other digestive disorders because of its antioxidant and anti-inflammatory properties, and it also helps increase the good bacteria in your gut. Cabbage not only assists in prevention of many types of cancers but for some types is also used in their treatment.

Cayenne Pepper

- **Color:** Red

- **Yield:** If using fresh, 1 pound = 1 cup juice; using powder is also acceptable

- **Flavor Profile:** Extra spicy and rich

- **Health Benefits:** Cayenne pepper is a good source of antioxidants and, to a lesser extent, vitamin A. The capsaicin in peppers is a powerful tool used to treat ulcers, maintain cardiovascular health, and promote weight loss. It's also good for draining congested sinuses and is a natural pain reliever.

Fennel

- **Color:** Green or milky

- **Yield:** 1 pound = 1 cup juice

- **Flavor Profile:** Peppery and bright

- **Health Benefits:** Fennel is strong in antioxidants and adds a fresh, peppery flavor to your juices. It's rich in phytonutrients, vitamins C and B3, potassium, manganese, phosphorus, magnesium, copper, iron, folate, and calcium. Research suggests that fennel can help shut down the signaling system that may stimulate cancer growth in your liver. It also helps you maintain good cardiovascular and colon health and keeps your immune system strong.

Garlic and Onions

- **Color:** Milky

- **Yield:** 1 pound = 1 to 1¼ cups juice

- **Flavor Profile:** Pungent and spicy

- **Health Benefits:** It would take another entire book to fully review all of the health benefits of garlic and onions, but perhaps most important are that they are fantastic sources of antioxidants as well as vitamins B6 and C, folate, potassium, manganese, and tryptophan.

  Garlic and onions keep your immune system strong to help you fight off colds, the flu, and disease; they promote digestive health, help your body metabolize iron, which is great for your blood, and kill bacteria in your mouth that cause gum disease. And the big benefit? The sulfides and antioxidants are extremely anti-carcinogenic and protect you from a wide range of cancers.

Ginger

- **Color:** Milky

- **Yield:** 1 pound = ½ to ⅔ cup juice

- **Flavor Profile:** Zesty and extremely spicy

- **Health Benefits:** The gingerol in ginger is not only a powerful anti-oxidant but actually stimulates apoptosis, or cell death, in ovarian cancer. For centuries ginger has been used to treat stomach upset and disorders such as motion sickness. Ginger strengthens your immune system and is also great for reducing the swelling and pain associated with arthritis.

Horseradish

- **Color:** Milky

- **Yield:** 1 pound = ½ cup juice

- **Flavor Profile:** Extremely spicy

- **Health Benefits:** Horseradish can add a deliciously spicy zing to your green juices and smoothies and contains nutrients, antioxidants, and anti-inflammatories that lessen arthritis pain and swelling, fight off colds and the flu, and battle cancer, just to name a few benefits. It's also excellent for respiratory and sinus issues and promotes good urinary health. And as an added bonus, it's great for your skin and for detoxification.

Jalapeño Peppers

- **Color:** Green

- **Yield:** 1 pound = 1 to 1¼ cups juice

- **Flavor Profile:** Extremely spicy

- **Health Benefits:** Just as with cayenne peppers, jalapeños are a great source of capsaicin, and since they're green, you're getting the benefits of chlorophyll as well. They're great for digestion, and if you don't use the seeds, you can greatly reduce the heat.

Zesty and Tart

Grapefruits, Lemons, and Limes

- **Color:** Pink, yellow, or green

- **Yield:** 1 pound = 1 to 1½ cups juice

- **Flavor Profile:** Sweet and tart

- **Health Benefits:** Tart citrus fruits are delicious and chock full of vitamins A, B, and C. They're terrific for your immune system, and the antioxidants destroy free radicals that cause cancers such as breast, colon, lung, stomach, and skin cancers. They also have the phytonutrient limonin that keeps cancer cells from growing. Citrus juice can also help prevent certain kidney stones by lowering your pH, and assists in lowering your bad cholesterol as well.

Lemongrass

- **Color:** Green

- **Yield:** 1 pound = ⅔ to 1 cup juice

- **Flavor Profile:** Grassy with lemony tones

- **Health Benefits:** Lemongrass is great for juicing or cleansing, because in addition to the other benefits of chlorophyll, it also boosts your immune system, eliminates toxins, improves your energy levels by increasing the oxygen level in your blood, and promotes healing throughout your body.

Tomatoes

- **Color:** Red

- **Yield:** 1 pound = 1 to 1½ cups juice

- **Flavor Profile:** Rich and, well, "tomatoey"

- **Health Benefits:** Tomatoes are fantastic for your health and also make a great base for creating a green juice with a familiar flavor profile. They're rich in vitamins A (including beta-carotene and zeaxanthin), B complex, C, E, and K, as well as the minerals copper, iron, magnesium, tryptophan, phosphorus, and potassium. And, yes, tomatoes have protein, too. They're excellent for keeping your eyes, heart, and bones healthy, plus the antioxidant alpha-tomatine interferes with the growth of prostate and lung cancer cells, and possibly breast and pancreatic cancer cells also.

Watercress

- **Color:** Milky

- **Yield:** 1 pound = ⅔ to 1 cup juice

- **Flavor Profile:** Peppery

- **Health Benefits:** This zesty plant is both tasty and good for you. It's a natural diuretic and its antioxidants protect you from cancer. It has also been used for centuries as a digestive aid, and it helps with respiratory issues by clearing your airway.

> **Did You Know?** *If you're taking certain medications such as chlorzoxazone, you should speak with your doctor prior to consuming watercress, because there may be an interaction.*

Herbs

Basil

- **Color:** Dark green

- **Yield:** 1 pound = 1 cup juice

- **Flavor Profile:** Bright and refreshingly spicy

- **Health Benefits:** Basil has the same nutrients as other leafy greens and adds an appetizing, familiar "spaghetti sauce" zing to your juice. It's currently being studied for its antibacterial properties, because it's suspected that basil can fight disease-causing bacteria that have become immune to mainstream antibiotics. Because it has such a strong flavor, be careful adding more than just a few leaves!

Cilantro

- **Color:** Dark green

- **Yield:** 1 pound = 1 cup juice

- **Flavor Profile:** Spicy and grassy

- **Health Benefits:** Cilantro carries the same health benefits as other leafy greens and also helps control your blood sugar, while decreasing bad (LDL) cholesterol.

> **Did You Know?** *Cilantro, also known as coriander, adds a flavor reminiscent of salsa to your juice, because it's the primary herb used in that recipe. Like basil, cilantro is being studied for its beneficial antibacterial properties.*

Dill

- **Color:** Green

- **Yield:** 1 pound = ¾ to 1 cup juice

- **Flavor Profile:** Sweet and spicy

- **Health Benefits:** Packed with antioxidants, calcium, and antibacterial and anti-inflammatory properties, dill is great for preventing osteoporosis, infections, heart disease, cancer, and other illnesses related to damage by free radicals. It's often used with chamomile to promote relaxation and sleep.

> **Did You Know?** *Dill has been used as a cure for hiccups and headaches for centuries. Just place it in boiling water, let it steep, drain, and drink the resulting tea.*

Mint

- **Color:** Bright green

- **Yield:** 1 pound = ⅔ to 1 cup juice

- **Flavor Profile:** Sweet, bright, and refreshing

- **Health Benefits:** For centuries, this delicious leaf—used to make candy as well as a digestive aid to calm upset stomachs—packs a huge health punch. It contains antioxidants that fight cancer and is packed with antimicrobial oils that kill bad bacteria such as salmonella, E. coli, and staph. Mint is also great for respiratory problems related to inflammation, such as allergies and asthma. This bright green herb does way more than just taste good!

Parsley

- **Color:** Bright green

- **Yield:** 1 pound = ⅔ to 1 cup juice

- **Flavor Profile:** Grassy and vibrant

- **Health Benefits:** Parsley contains all of the benefits of other leafy greens, as well as volatile oils that have been shown to slow down tumor formation, particularly in the lungs. It's also rich in flavonoids, or antioxidants that fight free radicals and reduce your chances of getting cancer, including colon cancer. In addition, parsley reduces your odds of contracting such diseases as diabetes, asthma, heart disease, and atherosclerosis.

Radishes

- **Color:** Milky and the greens are, of course, green

- **Yield:** 1 pound = 2/3 to 1 cup juice

- **Flavor Profile:** Peppery and spicy; the greens are earthy and grassy with a hint of spice

- **Health Benefits:** The biggest thing radishes have going for them is their vitamin C content; they also contain trace minerals, though not in significant amounts. The vitamin C is a great detoxifier and can help protect you from several types of cancer, including oral, kidney, and digestive cancers. And as we all know, vitamin C is great for fighting off colds and the flu, as well as diabetes, cardiovascular disease, urinary tract infections, and kidney disease.

Spices

Cinnamon

- **Color:** Red or brown

- **Yield:** Use store-bought powder or freshly grind a stick at home

- **Flavor Profile:** Spicy and woodsy

- **Health Benefits:** This aromatic herb that reminds many people of the holidays is packed with antioxidants and anti-inflammatories that help you maintain heart, colon, and immune health. It also helps regulate your metabolism and blood sugar levels and is a natural antibacterial and anti-fungal. Throw cinnamon into your juice for a healthy burst of flavor!

Cloves

- **Color:** Brown

- **Yield:** Use store-bought powder or dried whole cloves

- **Flavor Profile:** Spicy, sweet, and woodsy

- **Health Benefits:** Cloves contain more antioxidants than any other ingredient, and therefore constitute an amazing addition to your juices. They blend well with both ginger and cinnamon, so feel free to throw them into drinks in which you're using those spices, too. Cloves also have antiseptic, anti-inflammatory, and germicidal properties, so they're great for heading off the flu, infections, arthritis, and digestive issues. Because of their high antioxidant content, cloves help your body fight everything from colds to cancer, so use them liberally!

Turmeric Root

- **Color:** Bright orange

- **Yield:** The actual root is pretty hard to find fresh, so just use it in powder form

- **Flavor Profile:** Spicy and slightly ginger-like

- **Health Benefits:** The benefits of this orange cousin of ginger are about as long as your arm, so we'll just touch on the most important ones. Turmeric doesn't just fight free radicals to prevent cancer, it actually blocks the enzyme that promotes its growth. It may also be useful in the actual treatment of certain cancers, including colon, prostate, and skin cancers. It's an amazing anti-inflammatory as well and is therefore beneficial to those with arthritis.

Other healthful and tasty additions to your juice include: honey, unwashed sea salt, black pepper, allspice, thyme, flaxseed, chia seeds, and oregano. This is only a list of some of the most popular fruits, vegetables, herbs, and spices. Just because something is not on the list doesn't mean that you can't use it or that it won't be good.

We've talked about the benefits of incorporating juice into your daily diet, but what if you want to cleanse and detoxify your body by undergoing a green juice cleanse? It's true that this is more drastic and can have some significant side effects, but if done properly, a good cleanse can really get your body back on track. In the next chapter, we'll discuss how to properly undergo a cleanse, what the health benefits are, and what potential side effects to expect.

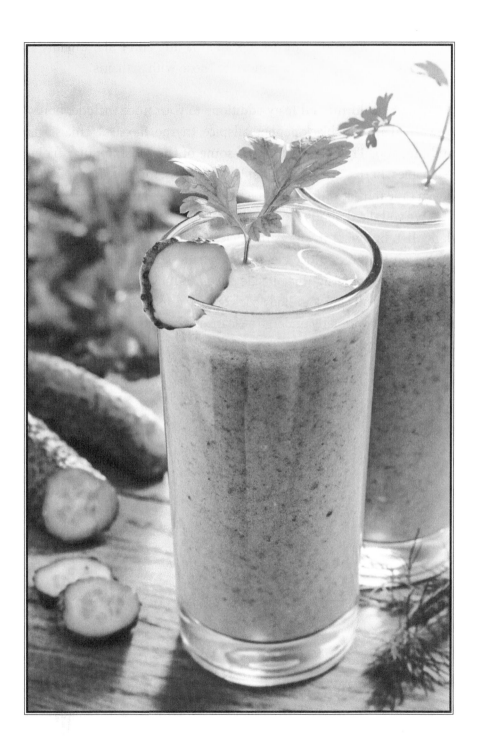

WHAT'S THE BIG DEAL ABOUT JUICE CLEANSING AND IS IT RIGHT FOR YOU?

Juice cleansing, also known as juice fasting, is exactly what it sounds like: eliminating everything except juice from your diet for a period of time in order to cleanse and detoxify your body. The problem is that many people fall in love with the idea of doing this but don't know how to properly prepare for the cleanse in order to be successful. Also, a cleanse is a major shock to your body, so there may be some pretty nasty side effects. By the end of this chapter, you will know exactly how to juice fast properly, enabling you to get the most out of your efforts.

What Are the Benefits of Fasting?

The first few days of a fast will be brutal, but the benefits of a juice cleanse are amazing. Not only will you feel better, but your body will be able to function better, too, which will improve your overall health in the long run. You probably aren't even aware of the toxins that your body is exposed to on a daily basis, but they're in the air you breathe, the water you drink, and the food that you eat. You can't escape them all, but you *can* take steps to cleanse your body of them periodically. Here are a few reasons why you should do so.

Immune System Boost and Healing

When your body gets bogged down from fighting the everyday toxins that you put into it, there's little time left for taking care of the business for which it was designed. When you stop putting in garbage, your body finally has time to mend all of the modest aches and pains that it shoved to the backburner in its effort just to keep you functioning. Because of this and other reasons, you may find that minor irritations such as muscle pain, niggling headaches, and heartburn disappear.

Healthy, Efficient Digestion

This one's a no-brainer, but it's a benefit many people don't consider because you don't realize how clogged up your digestive tract is until you start a juice cleanse. Once you've cleaned out your system, you'll likely find that gastric disorders such as gas, indigestion, and upset stomach that regularly plague you will disappear. There's nothing in there backing up the progress because your system is sparklingly clean and functioning the way it was intended!

Mental Clarity

Just about any doctor will tell you that brain function depends upon a healthy diet. What you put into your body is what you get out of it, and your brain requires certain nutrients just to shuttle messages back and forth. It's no surprise that when your system is clogged up with toxins, your nervous system is affected, too. Since your body is free of toxins after a cleanse and is receiving all that chlorophyll that helps with oxygen uptake, your brain is finally getting everything it needs to function optimally.

Increased Energy

Since your body is taking in a ton of nutrients, and your immune and digestive systems aren't working overtime, there will be plenty of energy left over, and you'll suddenly feel ten years younger! You may have thought that your get-up-and-go was gone, but get ready for a huge boost in your energy levels now that your body is free of toxins and functioning properly! As a matter of fact, this is one of the first "side effects" you'll notice and is a sure sign that your cleanse is working.

Amazing Skin

Your skin is going to thank you for your cleanse by looking brighter and being free of acne. It's a fairly well-known fact that one of the main causes of acne is a poor diet, but let's carry it a step further. Your body has only a few outlets for shoving out toxins, and your skin is one of them, so pimples are often an infection that your body is pushing out. When your body is free of toxins and receiving heaps of nutrients instead of junk, it's only logical that your skin will look amazing as a result.

Who Should Fast, and for How Long?

This is a great question because, for some people, fasting of any sort isn't healthy. If you're diabetic or are suffering from any major disease that requires a special diet, fasting probably isn't a good idea for you. Similarly, you may want to think twice about fasting if for any reason your immune system is already compromised. Even if you think that you're in great health, it's a good idea to discuss a juice fast with your doctor before you begin.

How long to fast is a personal decision. People who are fasting may do so for extended periods, or just for a day to give their bodies a quick break. Those who are simply cleansing tend to live on juice only for as long as they believe it takes to clear all the toxins from the body.

It takes two days or so for your body to clear all the fiber and other junk from your digestive tract, but after a week or so, your muscles start to deteriorate on juice alone, because you're not getting the protein you need to maintain and build them. The answer, then, is that you should fast for three to seven days in order to achieve optimal results without compromising your health.

Side Effects of Juice Cleansing

As we've already discussed, there are a few nasty side effects to juicing of which you should be aware. You know that saying about pain being weakness leaving the body? Well, that's kind of the same principle here. The side effects of cleansing are literally caused by poisons leaving your body, but after your system is cleared, you're going to feel incredible. Once all of the toxins are gone, and your digestive tract is free from years of accumulated junk, you'll feel like a new person—we promise!

Nausea and Vomiting

Since you're not slowing down the digestive absorption process with fiber, your body will get a huge burst of nutrients all at once. If it isn't used to fresh juice, the rush of nutrients may make you feel sick until you get used to this. It may help to dilute your juices by mixing them with an equal amount of water, at least for the first few days.

Headaches

It's likely that you'll experience a headache in the first few days of a cleanse, especially if you didn't wean yourself completely off chemical addictions such as caffeine. A headache is the main symptom of caffeine withdrawal but will go away after a couple days.

Breakouts, Bad Breath, and Body Odor

Your body has only so many means of releasing toxins, and your skin and the respiration process are two of the main channels. On the positive side, when you start to notice breakouts and bad breath, you'll know that your cleanse is working; on the negative side, all of the people around you will notice, too. Since it can actually get pretty bad during the first few days, you may want to take some time off from work or start your cleanse at the beginning of a three-day weekend.

Diarrhea or Constipation

Since you're not eating solid foods and don't have the fiber to slow things down, you may experience diarrhea until your body flushes all of the toxins out. If it gets too bad, add a bit of fiber back into your diet by eating some celery or a cucumber for a few days, as you don't want to become dehydrated. On the other hand, the general absence of fiber during the cleanse may cause you to go the other direction and experience some constipation. If so, try adding some prune juice or another natural laxative into your juice.

Lethargy

It's pretty typical to experience a sudden lag in energy for the first couple days of a fast, because you're not eating solid carbohydrates, sugars, caffeine, and other junk. The carbs that you're getting from juice are rapidly absorbed and used, so spikes of energy followed by crashes are also common. You should be fine after a few days though, once you've adjusted to the juice and the toxins have left your body.

Tips for a Successful Juice Cleanse

Now that you know approximately how long it takes to clean out your body, and you understand the benefits and side effects that you can expect from a juice cleanse, there are a few things that we'd like to share in order to make your cleanse more successful. After we review these tips, we'll get to the good stuff—the recipes!

Don't Give Up

The first few days of your juice cleanse will very likely be brutal, but remember, you wouldn't feel like this if your body weren't congested with toxins. Also, it helps to keep in mind that it's the toxins leaving your body that are causing all of the side effects—not the juice.

When your breath is foul and you smell terrible, imagine that the odor wafting from you is a cloud of toxic waste leaving your body, because it quite literally is. Once you think of it in these terms, it will be much easier for you to persevere, because you certainly don't want to leave that nastiness *inside* your body, do you?

Drink Plenty of Water

Because you're consuming so many pure nutrients, you need to drink enough water to ensure that you don't become nauseated while your body is adapting. You need equal parts water and juice to efficiently flush the waste and toxins from your body. You can either dilute your juice, or drink a glass of juice followed by a glass of water—whichever you prefer. If you like, you can also drink herbal tea or fortified water as long it contains no caffeine, artificial preservatives, or other such garbage.

Don't Use Too Many Fruits

We've already discussed the energy peaks and valleys you may experience because of the quick uptake of carbohydrates, so it's a good idea to use as few fruits as possible, since they have higher amounts of natural sugars than vegetables do. Also, fruits are typically used for energy, while vegetables usually have more healing and restorative properties. Since you're cleansing, detoxifying, and healing, vegetables are the best tools for a green cleanse. Try to limit fruit juices to breakfast only, and stick with vegetable juices (mostly green, if possible) for the rest of the day.

Did You Know? *Most store-bought juices are pasteurized, using heat to kill any bacteria, but this process kills beneficial enzymes as well. Since you're making juice from raw produce, try to use organic produce only, if at all possible, and be sure to wash your produce thoroughly before juicing it.*

Make Your Juice As You Go

The longer your juice is exposed to air, the more nutrients it loses. For instance, vitamin C is purported to break down at a rate of about 2 percent per day, even in an airtight, opaque container. As soon as your juice is exposed to air, the oxidation process begins, so if at all possible, make your juice as you consume it. If this isn't possible, follow the guidelines we've already discussed, such as storing juice in an airtight container in the refrigerator.

Wean Yourself Off Addictions in Advance

You may not think you have many addictions, but if you start your day with a donut, a cup of coffee, and a cigarette, you may want to wean yourself off the sugar, caffeine, and nicotine at least a week before you begin your cleanse. As a matter of fact, you may want to put away the cigarettes a few weeks prior to a juice cleanse for the sake of preserving your sanity.

Your body will have enough to adapt to when you switch to pure juice without going through chemical withdrawal as well. Save yourself some serious misery and cut out heavily processed foods, alcohol, cigarettes, and caffeine slowly before you start your cleanse.

Don't Cheat!

The purpose of a juice cleanse is obviously to *cleanse*. That means you're sweeping away all of the garbage large and small from your digestive tract as well as the rest of your body, allowing your immune system to heal all that ails you and letting your system function properly.

The idea behind juice cleansing is that a huge percentage of your daily energy consumption goes toward digestion; when you're not consuming foods that require digestion, your body can use that energy to heal. If you're still eating solid food, you're defeating the purpose of a cleanse. So dedicate yourself to doing it right, and stick with it!

These simple tips should help get you started should you decide to take on a juice cleanse. So now it's time to discuss some specific needs you may like to address by juicing, and provide you with some delicious recipes to set you on your way to a healthier, greener you!

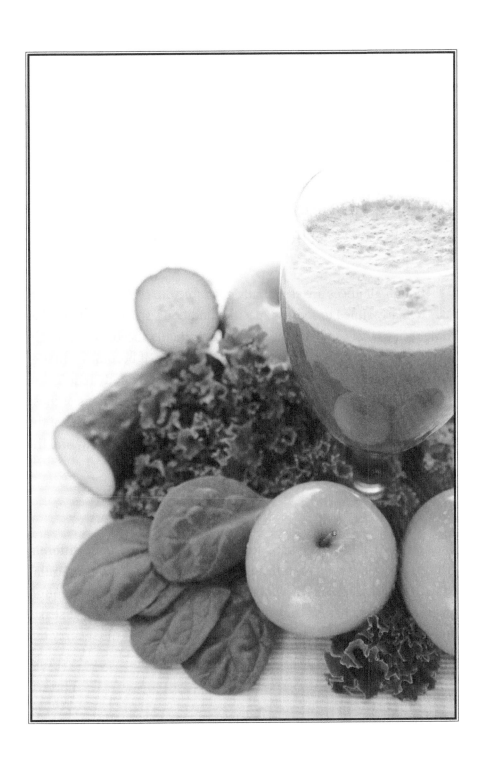

(6)

GREEN JUICE AND SMOOTHIE RECIPES TO CURE WHAT AILS YOU!

Though all juices are essentially good for you, certain ones are particularly suited to address specific conditions, so we've put together some recipes that can help you meet your particular needs. As we begin to understand how nutrients work in our bodies, it becomes a matter of finding the foods that contain the nutrients your body requires to fight off certain conditions, then eating the right combinations of those foods to give it the necessary tools to stay healthy. Here are some of the most common ailments that juices and smoothies can remedy and the great combinations you can try at home.

Detoxification

Because your body is exposed to toxins daily in dozens of different circumstances, it's important to detoxify your system on a regular basis. Drinking plenty of water helps, but it's simply not enough when your body has to continue to digest your food, fight disease, and perform the thousands of other functions that it must carry out for basic survival.

You need to clean your system periodically in order to maintain your good health, so here is a collection of recipes to get you started. The ingredients in the following recipes have been measured out for juice, so if you are making smoothies, decrease the measurements by about three-quarters.

Apple Juice Detox

This recipe is light and delicious but is also a cleansing powerhouse. Because of the high sugar content, this is a great breakfast juice to get your day started.

- ½ pound green apples
- ½ pound mint leaves
- 1 lemon
- 1 orange
- 1 cucumber

Process the apples and mint in a juicer, then the lemon and orange, followed by the cucumber. Stir well to combine. If using a blender, simply add all the ingredients (be sure to peel the lemon and orange first) and puree until smooth.

Yield: 12 to 14 ounces

Did You Know? *Apples have been used for centuries as a natural detoxifier due to their malic acid content. The lemon and orange may help dissolve certain types of kidney stones, and the vitamin C they contain serves to promote healing and fight free radicals.*

Dandy-Kale Delight

The rich green color of this drink gives you a sense of the healing benefits of its ingredients.

- ½ pound dandelion greens
- ½ pound kale leaves
- ¼ pound parsley
- 1 pound cucumber
- ½ pound celery

Process the dandelion greens, kale, and parsley in a juicer, then the cucumber and celery. Stir well to combine. If using a blender, simply add all the ingredients and puree until smooth.

Yield: About 20 ounces

Italian Fennel Cleanse

The fennel in this juice adds a peppery flair, and the lemon juice freshens it up, while everything works together to detoxify your body.

- ¼ pound garlic cloves, peeled
- ½ pound fennel
- ½ pound kale leaves
- 8 basil leaves
- ½ pound tomatoes
- ¼ pound cucumber
- 1 lemon

Process the garlic, fennel, kale, and basil in a juicer, then the tomatoes, cucumber, and lemon. Stir well to combine. If using a blender, simply add all the ingredients (be sure to peel the lemon first) and puree until smooth.

Yield: About 15 ounces

The Delicious Green Cleanse

This attractive green drink is as good for you as it looks. Fortunately it tastes refreshing and pleasant while working hard to fight diseases and detoxify your body. Each of the ingredients works well independently, but together they create a real powerhouse. If this drink tastes too rich, just add a little more cucumber.

- ½ pound green bell peppers
- ¼ pound broccoli florets
- ½ pound cucumber
- ½ pound cabbage

Process the bell peppers and broccoli in a juicer, then the cucumber and cabbage. Stir well to combine. If using a blender, simply add all the ingredients and puree until smooth.

Yield: About 14 ounces

Popeye's Pride

This rich green drink will really give your body a detoxifying boost. The lemon and celery work to cleanse while lending a refreshing taste to balance the spinach.

- 1 pound spinach
- 1 lemon
- ¼ pound parsley
- ½ pound celery

Process the spinach and lemon in a juicer, then the parsley and celery. Stir well to combine. If using a blender, simply add all the ingredients (be sure to peel the lemon first) and puree until smooth.

Yield: About 16 ounces

Weight Loss

Most vegetable juice blends are great for weight loss, especially the green ones. If you really want to amp up the race to slim down, try to stay as green as possible, because green usually indicates cleansing and low calories. Weight loss efforts can be thwarted by a sluggish metabolism, but cleansing your system can really help to rev up your internal energy furnace and get you closer to that svelte new you!

Cabbage Soup Juice

Rich in vegetables that help your body to detoxify and flush out toxins, this juice is both delicious and nutritious. Since it's so nutrient dense, you can actually fast on this juice for a few days if you choose to really cleanse your system.

- ½ pound green cabbage
- ¼ pound garlic cloves, peeled
- 6 to 8 basil leaves
- ½ pound tomatoes
- ½ pound green bell peppers

Process the cabbage, garlic, and basil in a juicer, then the tomatoes and bell peppers. Stir well to combine. If using a blender, simply add all the ingredients and puree until smooth.

Yield: About 12 ounces

Did You Know? *A powerful detoxifying agent and weight loss aid, cabbage makes a great base anytime you want to prepare a cleansing juice. The basil and green peppers are packed with chlorophyll, so you're getting good oxygen flow in addition to all of the health benefits of the other vegetables.*

Skinny Salsa Sauce

Made with many of the same vegetables found in salsa, this pleasant-tasting juice is low in calories and great for cleansing and detoxifying your entire system so that your metabolism functions efficiently. The large amount of chlorophyll increases your oxygen usage, enabling your body to drop unhealthy excess weight more quickly. Note: If your juicer can't handle the grasses, just leave them out.

- ¼ pound green onions
- ¼ pound wheatgrass
- ¼ pound lemongrass
- ¼ pound cilantro
- 1 pound tomatoes
- 1 lime

Process the green onions, wheatgrass, and lemongrass in a juicer, then the cilantro, followed by the tomatoes and lime. Stir well to combine. If using a blender, simply add all the ingredients (be sure to peel the lime first) and puree until smooth.

Yield: 16 to 20 ounces

Vegetable Soup Juice

Everybody who has ever tried to drop a pound—or twenty—has heard of the vegetable soup diet. This juice is a tasty play on that and is great for a mini-fast to kick-start your dieting efforts. The cayenne pepper gives it an extra metabolism-boosting kick.

- ¼ pound potatoes
- ¼ pound green onions
- 1 pound tomatoes
- ½ pound green bell peppers
- ¼ teaspoon black pepper
- Pinch of cayenne pepper

Process the potatoes and onions in a juicer, then the tomatoes and bell peppers. Add the black and cayenne peppers to the juice, and stir well to combine. If using a blender, simply add all the ingredients and puree until smooth.

Yield: About 20 ounces

Perfect Pepper Picker-Upper

This juice has an amazing peppery flavor, and the capsaicin it contains will really boost your metabolism.

- ½ jalapeño pepper
- ½ pound green bell peppers
- ½ pound cucumber
- ½ pound arugula

Process the jalapeño and bell peppers in a juicer, then the cucumber and arugula. Stir well to combine. If using a blender, simply add all the ingredients and puree until smooth.

Yield: About 16 ounces

Skinny Spaghetti in a Glass

This juice will remind you of a delicious spaghetti sauce because of the basil and tomato combination. It's a pleasant juice that will help keep you full, while providing a delightful burst of nutrition.

- ¼ pound garlic cloves, peeled
- ¼ pound green bell peppers
- 6 basil leaves
- 1 pound tomatoes

Process the garlic and bell peppers in a juicer, then the basil and tomatoes. Stir well to combine. If using a blender, simply add all the ingredients and puree until smooth.

Yield: About 12 ounces

Disease Prevention

In order to keep your body disease free, you need to do three important things on a regular basis. First, you should maintain a relatively alkaline environment, because diseases such as cancer can't grow under those conditions. Second, you need to keep your system clean, so your body can fight disease the way it's meant to do. Finally, give your body the nutrients it needs, such as antioxidants, to fight and prevent diseases on an ongoing basis. The following juices will help keep you on track for a disease-free existence!

Antioxidant Ale

This is a terrific juice to start off your day: the antioxidant punch is absolutely out of this world and so is the flavor! The fruit gives you a nice energy pop, too.

- ¼ pound raspberries
- ¼ pound oranges
- ¼ pound strawberries
- 4 mint sprigs, optional
- ¼ pound cucumber

Process all the ingredients in a juicer, and stir well to combine. If using a blender, simply add all the ingredients (be sure to peel the oranges first) and puree until smooth.

Yield: About 8 ounces

Super Shake

Help your body to prevent disease and stay nutrient-strong with "super" ingredients like garlic, kale, beets, and carrots. If you like, feel free to add a pinch or two of cayenne pepper to the mix for an extra antioxidant boost from the capsaicin.

- 1 head garlic, peeled
- ½ pound cabbage
- ½ pound kale leaves
- ½ pound beets
- ½ pound carrots
- ½ pound celery

Process the garlic, cabbage, and kale in a juicer, then the beets and carrots, followed by the celery. Stir well to combine. If using a blender, simply add all the ingredients and puree until smooth.

Yield: About 20 ounces

Did You Know? *Consuming lots of antioxidants is extremely important, but if you don't drink enough water to flush the free radicals, toxins, and disease from your body, the antioxidants can't effectively protect you!*

Thanksgiving in a Glass

This tastes so delicious you won't believe it's good for you, but rest assured—it is! The spices are fantastic antioxidants, and the apples and pumpkin contain all the vitamins necessary for disease prevention. This juice is also excellent for your eyes, so drink up!

- ½ pound green apples
- ½ pound pumpkin
- ½ pound cucumber
- ½ pound carrots
- ½ teaspoon ground cloves
- ½ teaspoon ground cinnamon

Process the apples and pumpkin in a juicer, then the cucumber and carrots. Add the cloves and cinnamon to the juice, and stir well to combine. If using a blender, simply add all the ingredients and puree until smooth.

Yield: About 16 ounces

Arugula Pepper Punch

This zesty drink is packed full of chlorophyll, cancer-fighting antioxidants, vitamins, and minerals. It also has a light, peppery flavor that's great for lunchtime.

- 1 pound arugula
- ¼ pound watercress
- ½ pound celery
- ½ pound lemongrass
- ¼ pound green bell peppers
- ½ teaspoon prepared horseradish

Process the arugula, watercress, and celery in a juicer, then the lemongrass and bell peppers. Add the horseradish to the juice, and stir well to combine. If using a blender, simply add all the ingredients and puree until smooth.

Yield: About 16 ounces

Rabbit Juice

This juice has a fairly green flavor, but its benefits are top-notch—you may just love it.

- 1 pound carrots
- ½ pound green apples
- ½ pound cucumber
- ½ pound kale leaves

Process all the ingredients in a juicer, and stir well to combine. If using a blender, simply add all the ingredients and puree until smooth.

Yield: About 20 ounces

Healthy Skin

It really is true that we are what we eat, so if you're not eating wholesome, healthy foods, your skin is going to reflect your poor dietary habits. If you'd like to clear up your complexion and have beautiful, glowing skin, these juices are formulated just for you!

Potato Head

Potatoes are often used as an alternative treatment for acne, and the vitamin A in tomatoes really helps your skin to glow. If you like, feel free to throw in some parsley, too.

- 1 pound potatoes
- 6 basil leaves
- 1 pound tomatoes

Process the potatoes and basil in a juicer, then the tomatoes. Stir well to combine. If using a blender, simply add all the ingredients and puree until smooth.

Yield: About 16 ounces

Green with Envy

Adding this drink to your juicing schedule a couple of times per week will have everyone pea green with envy over your beautiful complexion! The chlorophyll, antioxidants, and vitamins A and C in these vegetables will have your skin glowing in no time.

- ¼ pound broccoli florets
- ¼ pound cucumber
- ¼ pound kale leaves
- ¼ pound green bell peppers
- ½ pound tomatoes
- ½ pound celery

Process the broccoli, cucumber, and kale in a juicer, then the bell peppers and tomatoes, followed by the celery. Stir well to combine. If using a blender, simply add all the ingredients and puree until smooth.

Yield: About 16 ounces

See Your Way to Beauty Juice

This juice combines produce that's great for your skin and your eyes. After all, you want to be able to see how great your face looks, right? Plus it tastes great. If you like, toss in some cinnamon for an even more nutritious and flavorful kick!

- ½ pound carrots
- ½ pound cucumber
- ½ pound sweet potatoes
- ½ pound carrot greens
- ¼ pound arugula
- ¼ pound lemongrass

Process the carrots, cucumber, and sweet potatoes in a juicer, then the carrot greens and arugula, followed by the lemongrass. Stir well to combine. If using a blender, simply add all the ingredients and puree until smooth.

Yield: About 20 ounces

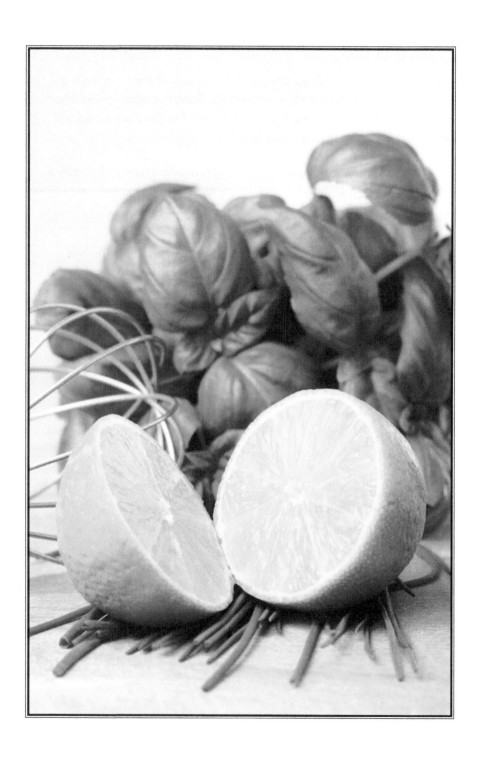

CONCLUSION

Throughout the pages of this book we've examined what green juices and smoothies are and the differences between the two. We've also touched on reasons why juices can be more beneficial for some purposes while smoothies meet other needs.

When it comes right down to it, both are excellent for your health and offer benefits that you'll start reaping almost immediately. Most people don't eat nearly their daily requirement of fruits and vegetables, and both juices and smoothies are great ways to give your body what it needs to function properly and keep you healthy.

Just to reiterate some of the most important things we've covered, here's a quick list:

- Use only fresh organic fruit whenever possible.
- Wash your produce thoroughly before using it.
- Drink your juice or smoothie immediately if at all possible.
- Eliminate bad habits such as smoking, drinking caffeine, or consuming large amounts of sugar at least two weeks prior to a cleanse.
- Consuming juices and smoothies isn't a diet—it's a habit to develop that helps you enjoy a lifetime of good health!

Now that you have a basic idea of how to make juices or smoothies, it's time to jump in! Remember the guidelines we've discussed for combining flavors, and always keep apples, cucumbers, lemons, and celery on hand to pull potentially disastrous experiments back from the brink. Practice makes perfect: Once you get comfortable throwing produce in the juicer or blender, you'll do just fine.

Cheers to great health!

CPSIA information can be obtained at www.ICGtesting.com
Printed in the USA
LVOW011222030613

336659LV00006B/14/P